21-Days

carb cycling:

Revitalize your body with balanced meals and effective workouts"

by

Julie J. Shively

Disclaimer

All rights reserved. No part of this publication may be reproduced, distributed, or transmitted in any form or by any means, including photocopying, recording, or other electronic or mechanical methods, without the prior written permission of the publisher, except in the case of brief quotations embodied in critical reviews and certain other noncommercial uses permitted by copyright law.

Copyright © **Julie J. Shively**, 2024

● **TABLE OF CONTENT**

Introduction

The morning sun filtered through the kitchen window, casting a golden glow over the countertops. Olivia stood there, looking at her reflection in the glass, feeling a mix of determination and apprehension. She had tried numerous diets before, each one promising miraculous transformations and each one leaving her more disheartened than the last. She needed something different, something sustainable, something that would not just change her body but also her life. That's when she discovered carb cycling. For years, Olivia had battled with her weight. From the latest fad diets to intensive workout regimes, she had seen it all. Each new approach began with a burst of enthusiasm, only to fizzle out as the days turned into weeks. It was during one of these periods of frustration that she stumbled upon the concept of carb cycling. Intrigued, she began to delve deeper, uncovering the science behind it and reading testimonials from those who had found success where she had only found failure. There was something different about carb cycling – it seemed to promise not just a diet, but a balanced lifestyle. Carb cycling is a dietary approach that alternates between high-carb and low-carb days to optimize fat loss and muscle gain. It's a method used by bodybuilders and athletes, but it's also accessible to anyone looking to revitalize their health and achieve sustainable weight loss. Unlike traditional diets that demonize entire food groups or drastically cut calories, carb cycling works with your body's natural rhythms and energy needs. The idea of carb cycling is simple yet powerful. On high-carb days, you fuel your body with the energy it needs for intense workouts and recovery, allowing your muscles to rebuild and grow stronger. On low-carb days, your body taps into stored fat for energy, promoting fat loss while preserving lean muscle mass. This dynamic approach not only keeps your metabolism revved up but also helps you avoid the plateaus that so often accompany conventional dieting. Olivia decided to give it a try. She started by setting realistic goals and armed herself with the knowledge she needed. She learned how to balance her macronutrients, understood the importance of hydration, and discovered how to pair her workouts with her dietary plan. Her kitchen became a laboratory of sorts, where she experimented with new recipes, and meals prepared for the week, and tracked her progress meticulously. The first week was challenging, as all new endeavors often are. There were moments of doubt, times when cravings threatened to derail her progress, and instances when she wondered if this would be just another failed attempt. But Olivia pushed through, motivated by the small victories – the extra energy she felt during her workouts, the slight loosening of her clothes, and the improvement in her mood and mental clarity. As the days turned into weeks, Olivia noticed significant changes. Her body began to respond positively to the carb-cycling regimen. She felt stronger, leaner, and more energized than she had in years. But beyond the physical transformations, there was something even more profound happening. She felt in control of her health and her life. This wasn't just another diet; it was a sustainable lifestyle change. This book is a culmination of Olivia's journey and the journeys of many others who have found success with carb cycling. It's designed to be your comprehensive guide to understanding, implementing, and thriving on a carb cycling plan. Whether you're a seasoned athlete looking to optimize your performance or someone who has struggled with weight loss for years, this book has something for you. In the pages that follow, you'll find detailed explanations of the science behind carb cycling, practical tips for meal planning and preparation, and a variety of delicious recipes tailored for both high-carb and low-carb days. You'll also discover effective workout routines that complement your dietary plan, helping you maximize fat loss and muscle gain. Most importantly, you'll learn how to overcome the common challenges that can arise on this journey, from dealing with cravings to staying motivated during tough times. The 21-Day Plan is at the heart of this book. This structured yet flexible program is designed to kickstart your carb cycling journey, providing you with daily meal plans and workout routines that are easy to follow and adapt to your lifestyle. Over three weeks, you'll build a foundation of healthy habits that will set you up for long-term success. Each week is carefully crafted to help you progress, keeping you motivated and engaged as you move towards your goals. Week One is all about getting started. You'll learn the basics of carb cycling, set up your kitchen for success, and begin to adjust to the new eating patterns. It's a week of discovery and adaptation, where you'll start to see the initial benefits of this dynamic approach to nutrition and fitness.

Week Two is where you'll build momentum. By now, you'll have a good grasp of the fundamentals, and you'll begin to refine your meal plans and workouts to suit your needs. This is a crucial phase, as it's when many people start to see significant changes in their bodies and energy levels. You'll find tips on staying motivated and pushing through any challenges that arise. Week Three is the final push, designed to help you finish strong. You'll be more confident in your carb cycling routine and ready to take on more advanced workouts and meal plans. This week will solidify the habits you've developed, ensuring that you're prepared to maintain your progress long after the 21 days are over. Throughout the book, you'll also find inspiring success stories from people who have transformed their lives with carb cycling. These real-life testimonials provide valuable insights and motivation, showing you that sustainable weight loss and improved health are within your reach.

In addition to the structured 21-Day Plan, the book offers plenty of resources to support you on your journey. From a glossary of terms to help you understand the key concepts to recommended reading and useful apps, you'll have everything you need to stay informed and motivated. The appendices also include measurement conversion charts and an index, making it easy to find the information you need when you need it. The journey to better health and fitness is not always easy, but with the right tools and mindset, it's entirely achievable. This book is more than just a guide; it's a companion that will support you every step of the way. By the end of these 21 days, you'll not only see changes in your body but also feel a renewed sense of confidence and well-being. You'll have the knowledge and skills to continue your carb cycling journey, making sustainable choices that benefit your long-term health. So, as you embark on this 21-day carb-cycling adventure, remember Olivia's story. Remember that every small victory counts and that perseverance will lead you to success. This is your opportunity to revitalize your body, transform your health, and reclaim your life. Welcome to the beginning of a new chapter – one filled with balanced meals, effective workouts, and the promise of a healthier, happier you.

Chapter 1: Understanding Carb Cycling: The Science Behind Carb Cycling

Carb cycling isn't just another fad diet; it's a strategic approach to eating that has roots in both sports nutrition and metabolic science. To truly understand carb cycling and its benefits, it's essential to delve into the science behind it, exploring how it works, why it works, and what makes it a sustainable method for weight loss and overall health improvement.

What is Carb Cycling?

Carb cycling is a dietary strategy that alternates between high-carb and low-carb days, to optimize the body's performance, metabolism, and fat-burning capacity. The primary goal is to time carbohydrate intake to maximize their benefits—fueling workouts and promoting muscle recovery—while minimizing their potential downsides, such as fat storage.This approach allows for flexibility and variation in your diet, which can prevent the monotony and deprivation often associated with strict dieting. By cycling carbs, you can enjoy the metabolic benefits of low-carb days while still having high-carb days to support energy levels and exercise performance

The Science Behind Carb Cycling

To understand the science of carb cycling, it's essential to grasp the fundamental roles of carbohydrates in the body. Carbohydrates are the body's preferred source of energy. When you consume carbs, they are broken down into glucose, which enters the bloodstream and is used by cells for energy. Any excess glucose is stored in the liver and muscles as glycogen.On high-carb days, you consume a higher amount of carbohydrates, which replenishes glycogen stores in the liver and muscles. This is particularly beneficial for high-intensity workouts and strength training, as glycogen is the primary fuel source for these activities. By ensuring your glycogen stores are full, you can perform better and recover more quickly. On low-carb days, carbohydrate intake is reduced significantly, forcing the body to utilize stored fat for energy. This shift in energy utilization promotes fat loss while preserving lean muscle mass. By alternating between high-carb and low-carb days, you can effectively balance muscle preservation and fat loss, which is a key advantage of carb cycling over traditional low-carb diets.

The Role of Insulin

Insulin, a hormone produced by the pancreas, plays a crucial role in carb cycling. When you consume carbohydrates, insulin is released to help cells absorb glucose from the bloodstream. Insulin is also known as an anabolic hormone, meaning it promotes the storage of nutrients, including glycogen in muscles and fat in adipose tissue.High-carb days stimulate insulin production, which aids in muscle recovery and growth by ensuring that muscles receive adequate glucose and other nutrients. Conversely, on low-carb days, insulin levels remain lower, which facilitates fat burning as the body turns to stored fat for energy.This strategic manipulation of insulin levels through carb cycling can help optimize body composition by promoting muscle gain on high-carb days and fat loss on low-carb days.

Types of Carb Cycling Plans

Carb cycling plans can vary significantly depending on individual goals, activity levels, and preferences. Here are a few common approaches:

1. Basic Carb Cycling: This involves alternating high-carb and low-carb days throughout the week. For example, you might have high-carb days on Monday, Wednesday, and Friday, and low-carb days on Tuesday, Thursday, and Saturday, with Sunday as a moderate-carb day.

2. Advanced Carb Cycling: This approach includes varying carb intake based on workout intensity. High-carb days coincide with intense workout days (e.g., leg days or high-intensity interval training), while low-carb days align with rest days or light activity days.

3. Keto Cycling: This is a variation that combines ketogenic (very low-carb) days with regular carb days. For example, you might follow a ketogenic diet for five days and then have two high-carb days to replenish glycogen stores.

4. Targeted Carb Cycling: In this approach, carbs are consumed around workout times (pre- and post-workout) to maximize performance and recovery, while the rest of the day remains low-carb.

The key to successful carb cycling is finding the right balance that works for your body and your lifestyle. It's important to listen to your body and adjust the plan as needed to achieve optimal results.

Benefits of Carb Cycling

Carb cycling offers several benefits beyond weight loss. Here are some of the most significant advantages:

1. Improved Metabolic Flexibility: By alternating between high-carb and low-carb days, you train your body to efficiently switch between using carbs and fats for fuel. This metabolic flexibility can enhance overall energy levels and improve performance in various activities.

2. Sustainable Weight Loss: Unlike restrictive diets that can be difficult to maintain, carb cycling provides a balanced approach that allows for flexibility and variety. This makes it easier to stick with the plan long-term and achieve sustainable weight loss.

3. Enhanced Muscle Preservation: By strategically timing high-carb days around intense workouts, you can support muscle growth and recovery while still promoting fat loss on low-carb days. This helps preserve lean muscle mass, which is essential for maintaining a healthy metabolism.

4. Hormonal Balance: Carb cycling can help regulate hormones, such as insulin, leptin, and ghrelin, which play critical roles in hunger, satiety, and energy balance. This can lead to better appetite control and reduced cravings.

5. Increased Energy and Performance: High-carb days provide the necessary fuel for intense workouts, improving exercise performance and recovery. This can help you achieve better results from your training and stay motivated to stay active.

6. Mental Health and Well-being: The flexibility and variety in carb cycling can reduce feelings of deprivation and improve adherence to the plan. This can lead to a more positive relationship with food and a greater sense of well-being.

Common Myths and Misconceptions

As with any dietary approach, carb cycling is subject to myths and misconceptions. It's important to separate fact from fiction to make informed decisions about your health and nutrition.

Myth 1: Carb Cycling is Only for Athletes

While carb cycling is popular among athletes and bodybuilders, it can be beneficial for anyone looking to improve their health and fitness. Whether you're an elite athlete or someone trying to lose weight and feel better, carb cycling can be tailored to meet your needs.

Myth 2: High-Carb Days Will Make You Gain Fat

The key to carb cycling is balance and timing. High-carb days are designed to replenish glycogen stores and support muscle recovery, not to promote fat gain. By combining high-carb days with appropriate workouts, you can ensure that the carbs are used effectively for energy and recovery rather than stored as fat.

Myth 3: Low-Carb Days Will Cause Muscle Loss

When done correctly, carb cycling preserves lean muscle mass. Low-carb days promote fat burning, but they are balanced with high-carb days that support muscle growth and recovery. Additionally, consuming adequate protein on low-carb days helps protect muscle tissue.

Myth 4: Carb Cycling is Complicated and Time-Consuming

Carb cycling may seem complex at first, but with proper planning and preparation, it can become a seamless part of your routine. By creating meal plans and preparing meals in advance, you can simplify the process and ensure you stay on track.

Myth 5: You Have to Give Up Your Favorite Foods

One of the advantages of carb cycling is its flexibility. While it's important to focus on whole, nutrient-dense foods, there's room for occasional treats and indulgences. The key is to incorporate them mindfully and in moderation, ensuring they fit within your overall plan.

How Carb Cycling Promotes Weight Loss

Carb cycling promotes weight loss through a combination of metabolic and hormonal mechanisms. Here's how it works:

1. Increased Fat Burning: On low-carb days, reduced carbohydrate intake forces the body to utilize stored fat for energy. This promotes fat loss while preserving lean muscle mass.

2. Optimized Glycogen Stores: High-carb days replenish glycogen stores, which supports high-intensity workouts and prevents muscle breakdown. This helps maintain muscle mass, which is crucial for a healthy metabolism.

3. Hormonal Regulation: Carb cycling helps regulate hormones like insulin, leptin, and ghrelin, which play critical roles in hunger, satiety, and energy balance. This can lead to better appetite control and reduced cravings.

4. Prevention of Metabolic Slowdown: Continuous low-carb dieting can lead to a slowdown in metabolism. By incorporating high-carb days, you can prevent this metabolic adaptation and maintain a higher metabolic rate, promoting sustained weight loss.

5. Increased Adherence: The flexibility and variety in carb cycling make it easier to stick with the plan long-term. This increases the likelihood of achieving and maintaining weight loss goals.

To get started with carb cycling, follow these practical tips:

1. Determine Your Caloric Needs: Calculate your daily caloric needs based on your goals, activity level, and body composition. This will help you determine how many calories to consume on high-carb and low-carb days.

2. Plan Your Meals: Create meal plans for high-carb and low-carb days, focusing on whole, nutrient-dense foods. Include a variety of protein sources, healthy fats, and fiber-rich vegetables to ensure balanced nutrition.

3. Track Your Progress: Keep a food journal or use a tracking app to monitor your carb intake and track your progress. This will help you stay accountable and make adjustments as needed.

4. Stay Hydrated: Proper hydration is essential for overall health and can support weight loss. Aim to drink at least 8 glasses of water per day, and more if you're active.

5. Listen to Your Body: Pay attention to how your body responds to carb cycling. Adjust your plan based on your energy levels, workout performance, and weight loss progress.

6. Be Flexible: Life happens, and there will be times when you need to adjust your

How Carb Cycling Promotes Weight Loss;Common Myths and Misconceptions

The Concept of Carb Cycling

Imagine a diet where you don't have to completely give up your favorite foods, where the flexibility of your meal plan keeps you motivated and satisfied, and where your body's metabolism works with you rather than against you. Welcome to carb cycling. At its core, carb cycling is a dietary approach that alternates between high-carb and low-carb days to maximize fat loss while preserving muscle mass and optimizing energy levels. It's a strategic and science-backed method to make dieting more effective and sustainable.

How Carb Cycling Promotes Weight Loss

Carb cycling promotes weight loss through a series of interconnected physiological processes. By understanding these mechanisms, you can appreciate why carb cycling is not just effective but also a more balanced approach compared to traditional diets.

1. Enhanced Fat Burning

On low-carb days, your body is deprived of its preferred energy source: glucose. As carbohydrate intake drops, the body shifts its primary energy source from carbohydrates to fats. This metabolic shift is known as ketosis, where the body begins to break down stored fat into fatty acids and ketones, which are then used for energy. This process helps reduce body fat over time.

Furthermore, the fluctuation between high and low-carb days prevents the body from fully adapting to one consistent low-carb state, which can lead to metabolic slowdown. By periodically reintroducing carbs, you keep your metabolism active and efficient at burning fat.

2. Optimized Glycogen Stores and Workout Performance

Glycogen, stored in muscles and the liver, is the body's readily available energy reserve for high-intensity activities. On high-carb days, the increased intake of carbohydrates replenishes these glycogen stores. This is particularly beneficial for athletes or individuals engaging in regular, intense workouts. Having adequate glycogen stores means you can train harder, longer, and more frequently, leading to greater calorie expenditure and muscle growth.

Muscle tissue is metabolically active, meaning it burns more calories at rest compared to fat tissue. By supporting muscle growth and recovery through high-carb days, you increase your resting metabolic rate (RMR), which can enhance long-term fat loss.

3. Hormonal Balance

Carb cycling has a profound impact on several key hormones involved in metabolism and weight management:

- **Insulin**: This hormone is critical for regulating blood sugar levels. On high-carb days, insulin levels rise to help store glucose as glycogen. Controlled insulin spikes can enhance muscle recovery and growth. On low-carb days, lower insulin levels help facilitate fat burning.

- **Leptin:** Known as the satiety hormone, leptin helps regulate hunger and energy balance. Long-term low-carb or calorie-restricted diets can decrease leptin levels, leading to increased hunger and reduced metabolic rate. High-carb days can boost leptin levels, helping to mitigate these effects and improve adherence to the diet.

- **Ghrelin:** Often referred to as the hunger hormone, ghrelin levels increase when you're hungry and decrease after eating. Carb cycling can help stabilize ghrelin levels by providing regular high-carb days that signal the body is not in a prolonged state of deprivation.

4. Prevention of Metabolic Slowdown

One of the significant challenges of long-term dieting is metabolic adaptation, where the body reduces its energy expenditure in response to a sustained calorie deficit. This is a natural survival mechanism designed to protect against starvation. By incorporating high-carb days, you periodically raise calorie intake, which can prevent or reduce the extent of metabolic slowdown. This "refeeding" strategy ensures your metabolism remains active, supporting ongoing weight loss.

5. Psychological and Behavioral Benefits

Traditional diets often fail because they are too restrictive and difficult to maintain over the long term. Carb cycling offers a psychological edge by providing regular high-carb days where you can enjoy a wider variety of foods. This can reduce feelings of deprivation, improve mood, and increase adherence to the diet. The anticipation of high-carb days can serve as a motivational tool, helping you stay committed on low-carb days.

Common Myths and Misconceptions About Carb Cycling

Like any popular diet trend, carb cycling is surrounded by myths and misconceptions. Addressing these can help you make informed decisions and maximize the benefits of this dietary approach.

Myth 1: Carb Cycling is Only for Athletes

While carb cycling is indeed popular among athletes and bodybuilders, it is by no means exclusive to them. This approach can benefit anyone looking to improve their health, manage weight, and enhance physical performance. The principles of carb cycling are versatile and can be adapted to suit various fitness levels, dietary preferences, and lifestyle needs. For example, someone who is moderately active might follow a simpler carb cycling plan with fewer high-carb days, while a highly active individual might incorporate more frequent high-carb days to support their training regimen. The key is customization and finding what works best for your unique circumstances.

Myth 2: High-Carb Days Will Make You Gain Fat

One of the most common fears about carb cycling is that high-carb days will lead to fat gain. This misconception arises from the misunderstanding of how the body processes carbohydrates. High-carb days are designed to replenish glycogen stores and support muscle recovery and growth. When timed correctly around physical activity, the carbohydrates consumed are used efficiently for energy and recovery, rather than being stored as fat. Moreover, the temporary increase in carbohydrates and calories can have positive effects on metabolism and hormone levels, which support long-term fat loss. The key is to maintain a balanced intake of macronutrients and to pair high-carb days with appropriate physical activity.

Myth 3: Low-Carb Days Will Cause Muscle Loss

There is a concern that reducing carbohydrate intake will lead to muscle loss, especially during low-carb days. While carbohydrates play a crucial role in muscle recovery and growth, the body can still preserve and build muscle with adequate protein intake and proper exercise. On low-carb days, it's important to prioritize protein to support muscle maintenance. Resistance training and strength exercises should also be incorporated to stimulate muscle growth and preserve lean tissue. The alternating nature of carb cycling ensures that muscle glycogen stores are periodically replenished, minimizing the risk of muscle loss.

Myth 4: Carb Cycling is Complicated and Time-Consuming

At first glance, carb cycling might seem complex and difficult to implement. However, with a little planning and preparation, it can become a straightforward and manageable part of your routine. The initial learning curve involves understanding your body's needs, calculating macronutrient ratios, and planning meals accordingly. Once you have a plan in place, meal prepping and scheduling high-carb and low-carb days can make the process easier. Utilizing tools like meal planning apps, food journals, and fitness trackers can help you stay organized and consistent. The flexibility of carb cycling also allows for adjustments based on your progress and lifestyle, making it a sustainable long-term approach.

Myth 5: You Have to Give Up Your Favorite Foods

One of the major advantages of carb cycling is its flexibility. Unlike restrictive diets that ban entire food groups, carb cycling allows you to enjoy a variety of foods, including your favorites, within the framework of high-carb and low-carb days. The key is moderation and timing. On high-carb days, you have the freedom to include foods that you might crave, such as pasta, bread, or even desserts, in a controlled manner. This helps reduce feelings of deprivation and makes the diet more enjoyable and sustainable. On low-carb days, focusing on nutrient-dense, whole foods can keep you satisfied and on track.

Myth 6: Carb Cycling is a Magic Bullet for Weight Loss

While carb cycling can be an effective tool for weight loss, it's not a magical solution. Successful weight management involves a combination of healthy eating, regular physical activity, adequate sleep, and stress management. Carb cycling works best when integrated into a balanced lifestyle that includes these other elements. It's also important to remember that individual responses to carb cycling can vary. What works for one person may not work for another, and adjustments may be necessary based on personal goals, preferences, and progress. Patience and consistency are crucial for achieving long-term success.

Implementing Carb Cycling

1. Assess Your Goals and Needs

Determine your primary goals, whether they are weight loss, muscle gain, improved athletic performance, or overall health. Consider your current activity level, dietary preferences, and lifestyle to tailor a carb cycling plan that suits you.

2. Calculate Your Macronutrient Needs

Calculate your daily caloric needs based on your goals and activity level. Use this information to determine your macronutrient ratios for high-carb and low-carb days. Typically, high-carb days involve higher carbohydrate intake with moderate protein and lower fat, while low-carb days involve higher protein and fat intake with reduced carbohydrates.

3. Plan Your Meals

Create meal plans for high-carb and low-carb days, focusing on whole, nutrient-dense foods. Ensure that your meals are balanced and provide adequate nutrients to support your goals. Meal prepping can save time and help you stay on track.

4. Schedule Your High-Carb and Low-Carb Days

Based on your activity level and workout schedule, plan your high-carb and low-carb days. High-carb days should coincide with intense workout days or days when you need extra energy. Low-carb days can be scheduled on rest days or light activity days.

5. Monitor Your Progress

Track your progress using a food journal, meal planning app, or fitness tracker. Monitor changes in weight, body composition, energy levels, and workout performance. Use this information to make necessary adjustments to your plan.

6. Stay Flexible and Adjust as Needed

Carb cycling is not a one-size-fits-all approach. Be open to making adjustments based on your progress and how your body responds. Listen to your body and modify your plan to ensure it remains effective and sustainable.

7. Prioritize Overall Health

Chapter 2: Preparing for Success

Achieving success with carb cycling requires more than just a basic understanding of the dietary strategy; it demands thorough preparation and a structured approach. In this chapter, we'll explore how to set realistic goals, equip your kitchen with essential tools and gadgets, and stock your pantry with the necessary staples to ensure you're always ready to stay on track with your carb cycling plan. This foundation will support your journey toward weight loss and improved health.

Setting Realistic Goals

Setting realistic, achievable goals is the first step in any successful endeavor. When it comes to carb cycling, your goals should be specific, measurable, attainable, relevant, and time-bound (SMART). Here's how to establish effective goals that will keep you motivated and on track.

1. Define Your Objectives

Begin by identifying your primary reasons for adopting a carb-cycling diet. Are you looking to lose weight, gain muscle, enhance athletic performance, or improve your overall health? Your objectives will shape your approach and help you tailor your plan to meet your specific needs.

2. Set Specific and Measurable Goals

Instead of vague goals like "lose weight" or "get fit," set specific targets. For example, "lose 10 pounds in three months" or "increase my bench press by 20 pounds in two months." Specific goals give you a clear direction and make it easier to track progress.

3. Make Your Goals Attainable

It's important to set goals that are challenging yet achievable. Setting unrealistic expectations can lead to frustration and demotivation. Consider your current fitness level, lifestyle, and time constraints when setting your goals. Achievable goals provide a sense of accomplishment and motivate you to continue.

4. Ensure Your Goals Are Relevant

Your goals should be relevant to your overall health and wellness objectives. Align your carb cycling goals with your broader health aspirations, such as improving energy levels, enhancing physical performance, or reducing body fat. This relevance keeps you focused and committed.

5. Time-Bound Goals

Assign a timeline to your goals to create a sense of urgency and a clear endpoint. Short-term goals (weekly or monthly) can keep you motivated, while long-term goals (six months to a year) help you stay focused on the bigger picture. For example, "lose 2 pounds per week" or "complete a 5K race in three months."

6. Track and Adjust

Regularly monitor your progress and be prepared to adjust your goals as needed. Use tools like food journals, fitness apps, or progress photos to keep track of your achievements. If you encounter setbacks, reassess your goals and make necessary adjustments to stay on course.

Essential Kitchen Tools and Gadgets

Equipping your kitchen with the right tools and gadgets can make meal preparation easier, more efficient, and more enjoyable. Here are some essential items to consider for a well-stocked kitchen that supports your carb-cycling plan.

1. Digital Kitchen Scale

A digital kitchen scale is invaluable for accurately measuring portion sizes and ingredients. Precise measurements help ensure you stay within your macronutrient targets and maintain consistency in your meals.

2. High-Quality Chef's Knife

A sharp, durable chef's knife is essential for efficient chopping, slicing, and dicing. Investing in a high-quality knife makes meal prep faster and safer.

3. Cutting Boards

Having multiple cutting boards for different food types (e.g., vegetables, meat, and fish) helps prevent cross-contamination and keeps your prep area organized. Opt for sturdy, non-slip cutting boards that are easy to clean.

4. Food Processor

A food processor can save you time and effort by quickly chopping, slicing, and shredding ingredients. It's particularly useful for preparing vegetables, making sauces, and creating homemade snacks.

5. Blender

A high-powered blender is perfect for making smoothies, soups, and sauces. It can also be used to blend protein shakes and other nutrient-dense beverages that are essential for meeting your nutritional needs.

6. Measuring Cups and Spoons

Accurate measurement tools are crucial for portion control and recipe consistency. A set of measuring cups and spoons ensures you can accurately measure dry and liquid ingredients.

7. Non-Stick Cookware

Non-stick pans and pots make cooking and cleaning easier. They allow you to cook with minimal oil, which can help reduce overall calorie intake. Invest in a high-quality set that includes a variety of sizes.

8. Meal Prep Containers

Reusable, airtight containers are essential for meal-prepping and storing food. Look for containers that are microwave and dishwasher-safe, and consider a variety of sizes to accommodate different portion sizes and meal types.

9. Slow Cooker or Instant Pot

A slow cooker or Instant Pot is perfect for preparing large batches of meals with minimal effort. These appliances are great for making soups, stews, and other dishes that can be portioned out for the week.

10. Water Filter Pitcher

Staying hydrated is crucial for overall health and weight loss. A water filter pitcher ensures you have access to clean, fresh water at all times, encouraging you to drink more throughout the day.

Stocking Your Pantry: Carb Cycling Essentials

A well-stocked pantry is the backbone of any successful dietary plan. Having the right staples on hand ensures you're always prepared to make nutritious meals that align with your carb cycling goals. Here are the essential items to include in your pantry.

1. Whole Grains and Starches

Whole grains and starches are the foundation of your high-carb days. They provide essential nutrients and sustained energy. Stock your pantry with:

- **Quinoa**

- **Brown rice**

- **Whole wheat pasta**

- **Oats**

- **Sweet potatoes**

- **Barley**

- **Bulgur**

These grains and starches can be easily incorporated into a variety of meals, from breakfasts to dinners.

2. Legumes and Beans

Legumes and beans are excellent sources of plant-based protein and fiber. They can be used in soups, salads, and main dishes. Keep a variety of dried or canned options, such as:

- **Lentils**

- **Chickpeas**

- **Black beans**

- **Kidney beans**

- **Pinto beans**

3. Protein Sources

Protein is essential for muscle maintenance and repair, particularly on low-carb days. Stock up on versatile protein sources such as:

- **Canned tuna or salmon**

- **Chicken breast (frozen or canned)**

- **Tofu and tempeh**

- **Greek yogurt**

- **Cottage cheese**

- **Protein powder**

Having a variety of protein options ensures you can create diverse and satisfying meals.

4. Healthy Fats

Healthy fats are important for satiety and overall health. Include a range of sources in your pantry:

- **Olive oil**

- **Coconut oil**

- **Avocado oil**

- **Nuts and seeds** (e.g., almonds, walnuts, chia seeds, flaxseeds)

- **Nut butter** (e.g., almond butter, peanut butter)

These fats can be used in cooking, baking, and as toppings for various dishes.

5. Low-Carb Vegetables

Vegetables are a key component of any balanced diet, providing essential vitamins, minerals, and fiber. Stock your pantry with a variety of low-carb vegetables that can be used in numerous recipes:

- **Leafy greens (e.g., spinach, kale)**

- **Broccoli**

- **Cauliflower**

- **Zucchini**

- **Bell peppers**

- **Cucumbers**

- **Tomatoes**

These vegetables can be eaten raw, steamed, roasted, or included in casseroles and stir-fries.

6. Herbs and Spices

Herbs and spices add flavor to your meals without extra calories. Keeping a variety of seasonings on hand ensures you can create delicious, flavorful dishes. Consider stocking:

- **Basil**

- **Oregano**

- **Thyme**

- **Rosemary**

- **Paprika**

- **Cumin**

- **Cinnamon**

- **Turmeric**

- Black pepper

Fresh herbs can also be kept in the fridge or grown in a small indoor garden.

7. Condiments and Sauces

Healthy condiments and sauces can enhance the taste of your meals. Look for options with minimal added sugars and preservatives:

- Low-sodium soy sauce

- Hot sauce

- Vinegar (e.g., balsamic, apple cider)

- Mustard

- Salsa

- Tomato paste

These condiments can be used to create marinades, dressings, and dips.

8. Whole Fruits

While fruit intake might be more controlled on low-carb days, it's still an important part of a balanced diet. Stock a variety of fresh and frozen fruits:

- **Berries (e.g., strawberries, blueberries, raspberries)**

- **Apples**

- **Bananas**

- **Oranges**

- **Grapes**

Frozen fruits can be added to smoothies or desserts, providing a convenient and nutrient-rich option.

9. Snacks

Healthy snacks are important for managing hunger and maintaining energy levels throughout the day. Keep a variety of nutritious options on hand:

- **Hummus and vegetable sticks**

- **Nuts and seeds**

- **Hard-boiled eggs**

- **Greek yogurt**

- **Protein bars (check for low sugar content)**

- **Air-popped popcorn**

These snacks can help you stay satisfied between meals and prevent overeating.

10. Hydration Essentials

Staying hydrated is crucial for overall health and weight loss. Keep these essentials in your pantry:

- **Herbal teas**

- **Green tea**

- Electrolyte packets or tablets (for high-intensity workout days)

- Infused water (add fruits, vegetables, or herbs to water for flavor)

Proper hydration supports digestion, energy levels, and overall well-being.

Preparing for Meal Planning and Prepping

Successful carb cycling requires consistent meal planning and prepping. Here's a step-by-step guide to help you get started:

1. Plan Your Weekly Meals

Take some time each week to plan your meals for both high-carb and low-carb days. Consider your schedule, workout plans, and food preferences. Write down your meal plan, including breakfast, lunch, dinner, and snacks.

Preparing for Success

Success in carb cycling doesn't happen by chance. It requires preparation, commitment, and a strategic approach to meal planning and progress tracking. In this chapter, we'll delve into the essentials of meal prepping, offering tips and tricks to streamline your efforts. We'll also explore effective methods for tracking your progress to ensure you stay on course and achieve your health and fitness goals.

Meal Prep 101: Tips and Tricks

Meal prepping is the cornerstone of any successful diet plan, and carb cycling is no exception. By preparing your meals in advance, you can ensure you stick to your nutritional goals, save time, and reduce the stress associated with daily cooking. Here's how to master the art of meal prep with practical tips and tricks.

1. Plan Your Meals

Start by creating a detailed meal plan for the week. Outline what you will eat for each meal on both high-carb and low-carb days. This plan should consider your personal preferences, nutritional needs, and schedule. Here's a step-by-step guide to effective meal planning:

- **Set Your Goals:** Define your macronutrient targets for high-carb and low-carb days. For instance, you might aim for 50% carbs, 30% protein, and 20% fat on high-carb days, and 20% carbs, 40% protein, and 40% fat on low-carb days.

- **Choose Your Recipes:** Select recipes that fit your carb cycling requirements. Look for variety to keep meals interesting and ensure a balance of nutrients.

- **Create a Shopping List:** Based on your meal plan, list all the ingredients you'll need. Group items by category (e.g., produce, proteins, grains) to streamline your grocery shopping.

2. Batch Cooking

Batch cooking involves preparing large quantities of food at once and dividing them into individual portions. This method saves time and ensures you have healthy meals ready to go. Follow these steps for efficient batch cooking:

- **Cook Staples in Bulk:** Prepare large batches of staple items like grilled chicken, quinoa, brown rice, roasted vegetables, and hard-boiled eggs. These can be used in various dishes throughout the week.

- **Invest in Quality Storage Containers:** Use BPA-free, airtight containers to store your meals. Glass containers are a great option as they are microwave and dishwasher safe.

- **Label and Date Your Meals:** Clearly label each container with the contents and date. This helps you keep track of freshness and avoid food waste.

3. Prep Ingredients in Advance

On days when you're too busy to cook, having pre-prepped ingredients can be a lifesaver. Spend some time prepping ingredients that can be quickly assembled into meals:

- **Wash and Chop Vegetables:** Clean and cut vegetables so they're ready to use in salads, stir-fries, or snacks.

- **Marinate Proteins:** Marinate meats or tofu in advance to enhance flavor and reduce cooking time.

- Pre-cook Grains and Legumes: Cook grains like rice and quinoa, and legumes like beans and lentils, and store them in the fridge for quick access.

4. Use Kitchen Gadgets

Leverage kitchen gadgets to simplify meal prep and reduce cooking time. Here are some must-have tools:

- **Slow Cooker/Instant Pot:** These appliances allow for hands-off cooking. Use them to prepare soups, stews, and large cuts of meat.

- **Blender/Food Processor:** Great for making smoothies, sauces, and chopping vegetables.

- **Air Fryer:** An air fryer can cook food quickly with minimal oil, perfect for making healthy versions of your favorite fried foods.

5. Portion Control

Portion control is crucial for maintaining your macronutrient targets. Use these strategies to ensure you're eating the right amounts:

- **Use Measuring Tools:** Invest in a good set of measuring cups, spoons, and a digital kitchen scale to accurately portion your food.

- **Pre-portion Snacks:** Divide snacks into individual servings. This prevents overeating and makes it easy to grab a healthy snack on the go.

- **Mindful Eating:** Pay attention to your hunger and fullness cues. Avoid distractions while eating to better gauge when you're satisfied.

6. Vary Your Menu

Eating the same meals every day can lead to boredom and make it harder to stick to your plan. Introduce variety by rotating different proteins, vegetables, and grains. Experiment with new recipes and spices to keep things interesting.

7. Stay Organized

Keep your kitchen and pantry organized to streamline meal prep. Here are some tips:

- **Arrange Your Pantry:** Keep similar items grouped and place frequently used items within easy reach.

- **Label Your Spices and Containers:** Use labels to quickly find what you need.

- **Maintain a Clean Workspace:** Clean as you go to keep your kitchen tidy and make cooking more enjoyable.

8. Be Flexible

While planning is essential, it's also important to be flexible. Life can be unpredictable, so have backup options like frozen meals or quick, healthy snacks available. If you miss a meal or have an unexpected event, don't stress. Simply get back on track with your next meal.

Tracking Your Progress

Tracking your progress is vital to understanding how your body responds to carb cycling and making necessary adjustments to your plan. Here are effective methods and tools for monitoring your journey.

1. Keep a Food Journal

A food journal helps you stay accountable and aware of what you're eating. Record everything you consume, including portion sizes, macronutrient breakdown, and timing of meals. This detailed log can reveal patterns, identify areas for improvement, and help you stay on track.

2. Use Apps and Technology

Leverage technology to simplify tracking. There are numerous apps designed to help you monitor your diet and progress:

- **MyFitnessPal:** This app allows you to log your food intake, track macronutrients, and set specific goals for high-carb and low-carb days.

- **Lose It!:** Another popular app for tracking calories and macros, with a large database of foods and a barcode scanner for easy entry.

- **Cronometer:** Provides detailed nutrient tracking, including vitamins and minerals, helping you ensure a well-rounded diet.

3. Monitor Physical Changes

Physical changes can be a more tangible indicator of progress than the number on the scale. Here are some ways to track these changes:

- **Measurements:** Use a tape measure to track changes in your waist, hips, chest, arms, and thighs. Take measurements every two weeks to monitor your progress.

- **Progress Photos:** Take photos from different angles (front, side, back) at regular intervals. Comparing these photos over time can visually demonstrate your progress.

- **Body Composition Analysis:** Consider using tools like a body fat scale or getting a professional body composition analysis to track changes in muscle mass and fat percentage.

4. Track Exercise and Performance

Recording your workouts and performance can provide insight into how carb cycling is impacting your fitness:

- **Workout Log:** Keep a log of your workouts, including the type of exercise, duration, intensity, and how you felt. Note any improvements in strength, endurance, or recovery.

- **Performance Metrics:** Track specific metrics relevant to your fitness goals, such as lifting weights, running times, or flexibility improvements.

5. Regular Check-ins

Regular check-ins help you stay accountable and make necessary adjustments. Schedule weekly or bi-weekly check-ins to review your progress:

- **Review Your Journal:** Look for patterns or trends in your food intake, energy levels, and physical changes.

- **Adjust Your Plan:** Based on your findings, make adjustments to your carb cycling plan. This could mean altering macronutrient ratios, changing meal timing, or modifying your workout routine.

- **Set New Goals:** As you achieve your initial goals, set new ones to keep yourself motivated and moving forward.

6. Listen to Your Body

Your body provides valuable feedback. Pay attention to how you feel and adjust accordingly:

- **Energy Levels:** Note how your energy fluctuates in a day and on different carb cycling phases. Adjust your intake if you're feeling consistently fatigued.

- **Hunger and Satiety:** Monitor your hunger levels and satisfaction after meals. Adjust portion sizes and macronutrient ratios to better manage hunger.

- **Mood and Mental Clarity:** Track how your diet impacts your mood and cognitive function. Ensure you're getting a balance of nutrients to support overall well-being.

7. Seek Support

Having a support system can greatly enhance your success. Consider these options:

- **Join a Community:** Online forums, social media groups, and local fitness clubs can provide support, motivation, and shared experiences.

- **Work with a Professional:** A dietitian, nutritionist, or personal trainer can offer personalized guidance, monitor your progress, and help you make informed adjustments.

8. Celebrate Your Successes

Recognize and celebrate your achievements, no matter how small. This positive reinforcement helps maintain motivation and commitment:

- **Set Milestones:** Break your larger goals into smaller milestones and celebrate each one you reach.

- **Reward Yourself:** Treat yourself to non-food rewards, such as new workout gear, a massage, or a fun outing.

9. Reflect and Reevaluate

Periodically reflect on your journey and reevaluate your goals. This process ensures you stay aligned with your long-term objectives and remain flexible in your approach:

- **Reflect on Your Journey:** Consider what's working well and what challenges you've faced. Use these insights to refine your strategy.

- **Reevaluate Goals:** As you progress, your goals may evolve. Regularly revisit and adjust your goals to stay motivated.

Chapter 3: Nutrition Fundamentals

Understanding the fundamentals of nutrition is crucial for any successful diet plan, especially one as nuanced as carb cycling. This chapter delves into the essential aspects of nutrition, explaining macronutrients—carbohydrates, proteins, and fats—and their roles in your diet. Grasping these concepts will enable you to make informed choices and tailor your carb-cycling strategy to meet your specific health and fitness goals.

Macronutrients Explained: Carbs, Proteins, and Fats

Macronutrients are the nutrients your body needs in large amounts to function properly. They provide energy, support bodily functions, and contribute to overall health. There are three primary macronutrients: carbohydrates, proteins, and fats. Each plays a unique role in your body, and balancing them is key to optimizing health and performance.

1. Carbohydrates

Carbohydrates are the body's primary energy source. They are found in a variety of foods, including fruits, vegetables, grains, and legumes. Carbohydrates can be classified into three main categories:

- **Sugars:** Simple carbohydrates, such as glucose, fructose, and sucrose, are found in fruits, vegetables, and sweeteners.

- **Starches:** Complex carbohydrates found in grains, legumes, and starchy vegetables like potatoes and corn.

- **Fiber:** Indigestible carbohydrates found in plant-based foods, which aid in digestion and promote gut health.

Functions of Carbohydrates:

- **Energy Production:** Carbs are broken down into glucose, which is used by cells for energy. They are especially important for high-intensity activities.

- Brain Function: The brain relies on glucose for energy. Adequate carbohydrate intake supports cognitive functions and mental clarity.

- Muscle Glycogen Storage: Carbs are stored as glycogen in muscles and the liver, providing a readily available energy source during physical activity.

- Gut Health: Fiber-rich carbs promote healthy digestion and prevent constipation by adding bulk to stool and supporting beneficial gut bacteria.

2. Proteins

Proteins are essential for building and repairing tissues, producing enzymes and hormones, and supporting immune function. They are composed of amino acids, which are categorized into essential and non-essential amino acids.

- Essential Amino Acids: These cannot be synthesized by the body and must be obtained through diet. Sources include animal products like meat, eggs, and dairy, as well as plant-based sources like beans, lentils, and quinoa.

- **Non-Essential Amino Acids:** These can be synthesized by the body. They are still important but do not need to be consumed in large quantities.

Functions of Proteins:

- **Muscle Growth and Repair:** Proteins are critical for muscle development and recovery, making them essential for athletes and active individuals.

- **Enzyme and Hormone Production:** Proteins are involved in the production of enzymes and hormones that regulate various bodily functions.

- **Immune Function:** Proteins contribute to the creation of antibodies, which are vital for immune defense.

- **Transport and Storage:** Proteins help transport nutrients and other molecules throughout the body and play a role in storing nutrients.

3. Fats

Fats are a concentrated source of energy and are vital for various bodily functions. They can be categorized into three main types:

- **Saturated Fats:** Found in animal products and some plant oils, these fats are solid at room temperature.

- **Unsaturated Fats:** Found in nuts, seeds, fish, and plant oils, these fats are liquid at room temperature and are further divided into monounsaturated and polyunsaturated fats.

- **Trans fats are found in some processed foods, these fats are artificially created and are associated with negative health effects.**

Functions of Fats:

- **Energy Storage:** Fats provide a dense source of energy, with each gram providing nine calories, compared to four calories per gram for carbs and proteins.

- **Cell Structure:** Fats are essential components of cell membranes, providing structural integrity and fluidity.

- **Hormone Production:** Fats are involved in the production of hormones, including sex hormones and cortisol.

- **Nutrient Absorption:** Fats aid in the absorption of fat-soluble vitamins (A, D, E, and K) and other essential nutrients.

- **Protection and Insulation:** Fats provide cushioning for organs and insulation to help regulate body temperature.

Balancing these macronutrients is crucial for maintaining health, optimizing performance, and achieving specific fitness goals.

The Role of Carbs in Your Diet

Carbohydrates often get a bad rap in the dieting world, but they play a critical role in a balanced diet, especially for those engaging in regular physical activity. Understanding the various functions and types of carbohydrates can help you incorporate them effectively into your carb cycling plan.

1. Carbs as a Primary Energy Source

Carbohydrates are the most readily available energy source for the body. When you eat carbs, they are broken down into glucose, which is either used immediately for energy or stored as glycogen in the liver and muscles for later use. This quick availability makes carbs particularly important for:

- **High-Intensity Exercise:** Activities like running, weightlifting, and sprinting rely heavily on glycogen stores. Carbs ensure you have the energy to perform at your best.

- **Brain Function:** The brain consumes about 20% of your daily energy intake, predominantly from glucose. Adequate carbohydrate intake is essential for maintaining cognitive function and mental clarity.

2. Carbs for Muscle Recovery and Growth

Post-exercise, your body needs to replenish glycogen stores and repair muscle tissue. Consuming carbohydrates along with protein after a workout can enhance recovery by:

- **Refilling Glycogen Stores:** Carbs help restore muscle glycogen levels, ensuring you have energy for your next workout.

- **Enhancing Protein Synthesis:** Carbohydrates trigger the release of insulin, a hormone that facilitates the uptake of amino acids into muscle cells, promoting muscle repair and growth.

3. Types of Carbohydrates

Not all carbs are created equal. Understanding the different types of carbohydrates can help you make healthier choices:

- **Simple Carbohydrates:** Found in sugary foods and drinks, simple carbs are quickly digested and provide a rapid energy boost. However, they can lead to blood sugar spikes and crashes.

- **Complex Carbohydrates:** Found in whole grains, legumes, and vegetables, complex carbs are digested more slowly, providing a steady release of energy and keeping you fuller for longer.

- **Fiber:** A type of carbohydrate that the body cannot digest. Fiber aids in digestion helps control blood sugar levels, and supports heart health. There are two types of fiber:

- **Soluble Fiber:** Dissolves in water and can help lower glucose and cholesterol levels. Found in oats, fruits, and legumes.

- **Insoluble Fiber:** Adds bulk to stool and helps food pass more quickly through the digestive tract. Found in whole grains, nuts, and vegetables.

4. Balancing Carbs in Your Diet

To optimize your carb intake for health and performance, consider the following strategies:

- **Focus on Whole Foods:** Prioritize whole, unprocessed foods like fruits, vegetables, whole grains, and legumes over refined carbohydrates like white bread, pastries, and sugary drinks.

- **Match Intake to Activity Level:** Adjust your carb intake based on your activity level. On days with intense workouts, increase your carb intake to fuel performance and recovery. On rest days or light activity days, reduce your carb intake to match your lower energy needs.

- **Distribute Carbs Throughout the Day:** Spread your carb intake across meals and snacks to maintain stable blood sugar levels and consistent energy throughout the day.

- **Consider Timing:** For optimal performance and recovery, consume carbs before and after workouts. Pre-workout carbs provide the energy needed for exercise, while post-workout carbs help replenish glycogen stores and support muscle recovery.

5. Carbs and Health

Beyond energy and performance, carbohydrates play a crucial role in overall health:

- **Heart Health:** Diets rich in whole grains, fruits, and vegetables (all good sources of complex carbs and fiber) are associated with a lower risk of heart disease.

- **Digestive Health:** Fiber-rich carbs support healthy digestion by promoting regular bowel movements and preventing constipation.

- **Blood Sugar Control:** Choosing low-glycemic index (GI) carbs, which are digested slowly, can help maintain stable blood sugar levels and reduce the risk of type 2 diabetes.

6. Myths and Misconceptions about Carbs

Despite their importance, carbohydrates are often misunderstood. Here are some common myths and the truths behind them:

- **Myth: All Carbs Are Bad:** The truth is, not all carbs are created equal. While refined carbs and sugary foods can contribute to health issues, complex carbs from whole foods are essential for health and performance.

- **Myth: Carbs Make You Fat:** Weight gain occurs when you consume more calories than you burn, regardless of the macronutrient. Carbohydrates themselves do not cause weight gain when consumed as part of a balanced diet.

- **Myth: You Should Avoid Carbs to Lose Weight:** While low-carb diets can be effective for weight loss, they are not the only approach. Balancing carbs with proteins and fats, and focusing on portion control, can also lead to successful weight loss.

Chapter 4: Meal Planning and Recipes

Embarking on a carb cycling journey requires meticulous meal planning to ensure you meet your nutritional needs while adhering to the principles of carb cycling. This chapter will guide you through creating balanced meal plans, provide sample meal plans for high-carb and low-carb days, and offer a variety of recipes for breakfast, lunch, dinner, snacks, and smoothies. Additionally, you will find tips for dining out while maintaining your carb cycling regimen.

How to Create a Balanced Meal Plan

Creating a balanced meal plan involves considering your macronutrient needs, meal timing, and variety to ensure you receive all essential nutrients while enjoying your meals.

Here's a step-by-step guide to help you design a meal plan tailored to your carb-cycling goals:

1. Determine Your Macronutrient Needs

Your macronutrient needs depend on various factors, including your age, sex, weight, activity level, and fitness goals. Carb cycling involves alternating between high-carb and low-carb days, so it's essential to calculate your macronutrient ratios for each day:

- **High-Carb Days:** Focus on higher carbohydrate intake to replenish glycogen stores and fuel intense workouts. Typically, 50-60% of your daily calories should come from carbohydrates, 25-30% from protein, and 15-25% from fats.

- **Low-Carb Days:** Reduce carbohydrate intake to promote fat burning while maintaining sufficient protein and fat intake. Aim for 20-30% of your daily calories from carbohydrates, 35-45% from protein, and 30-40% from fats.

2. Plan Your Meals and Snacks

Distribute your macronutrient intake across three main meals and 1-2 snacks per day. Ensure each meal includes a balance of protein, carbohydrates, and fats, tailored to whether it's a high-carb or low-carb day. Include a variety of foods to cover all essential vitamins and minerals.

3. Incorporate a Variety of Foods

Variety is key to preventing nutrient deficiencies and keeping your meals interesting. Rotate different protein sources (meat, fish, plant-based), carbohydrates (whole grains, fruits, vegetables), and fats (nuts, seeds, oils) throughout the week.

4. Prepare in Advance

Meal prep can save time and ensure you stay on track with your carb cycling plan. Cook and portion out meals ahead of time, store them in the fridge or freezer, and use airtight containers to keep them fresh.

5. Adjust Based on Feedback

Listen to your body and adjust your meal plan based on your energy levels, workout performance, and satiety. Keep a food journal to track your intake and make necessary modifications.

Sample Meal Plans for High-Carb and Low-Carb Days

Below are sample meal plans for high-carb and low-carb days to help you get started. Adjust portion sizes and ingredients based on your individual needs and preferences.

High-Carb Day Meal Plan

Breakfast: Greek Yogurt Parfait

- 1 cup Greek yogurt

- 1/2 cup granola

- 1/2 cup mixed berries

- 1 tablespoon honey

Snack: Apple with Almond Butter

- 1 apple, sliced

- 2 tablespoons almond butter

Lunch: Quinoa and Chickpea Salad

- 1 cup cooked quinoa

- 1/2 cup chickpeas

- 1/4 cup diced cucumbers

- 1/4 cup cherry tomatoes

- 2 tablespoons feta cheese

- 1 tablespoon olive oil

- 1 tablespoon lemon juice

Snack: Hummus and Veggie Sticks

- 1/2 cup hummus

- Assorted vegetable sticks (carrots, celery, bell peppers)

Dinner: Baked Salmon with Sweet Potato and Asparagus

- 6 oz baked salmon

- 1 medium sweet potato, baked

- 1 cup roasted asparagus

- 1 tablespoon olive oil

Low-Carb Day Meal Plan

Breakfast: Spinach and Mushroom Omelette

- 3 eggs

- 1 cup spinach

- 1/2 cup mushrooms, sliced

- 1/4 cup shredded cheese

Snack: Greek Yogurt with Chia Seeds

- 1 cup Greek yogurt

- 1 tablespoon chia seeds

Lunch: Grilled Chicken Salad

- 4 oz grilled chicken breast

- Mixed greens

- 1/4 cup cherry tomatoes

- 1/4 avocado, sliced

- 2 tablespoons olive oil

- 1 tablespoon balsamic vinegar

Snack: Cheese and Nuts

- 1 oz cheese (cheddar, mozzarella)

- 1/4 cup mixed nuts

Dinner: Beef Stir-Fry with Broccoli and Bell Peppers

- 6 oz lean beef strips

- 1 cup broccoli florets

- 1/2 cup bell peppers, sliced

- 2 tablespoons soy sauce

- 1 tablespoon olive oil

Breakfast Recipes

High-Carb Breakfast Options

1. Oatmeal with Banana and Peanut Butter

- Ingredients:

- 1/2 cup rolled oats

- 1 cup water or milk

- 1 banana, sliced

- 1 tablespoon peanut butter

- 1 teaspoon honey

- 1/2 teaspoon cinnamon

- Instructions:

1. Cook oats in water or milk according to package instructions.

2. Stir in peanut butter and honey.

3. Top with banana slices and sprinkle with cinnamon.

2. Smoothie Bowl

- Ingredients:

- 1 banana, frozen

- 1/2 cup mixed berries, frozen

- 1/2 cup Greek yogurt

- 1/2 cup almond milk

- Toppings: granola, chia seeds, fresh berries

- Instructions:

1. Blend frozen banana, mixed berries, Greek yogurt, and almond milk until smooth.

2. Pour into a bowl and top with granola, chia seeds, and fresh berries.

Low-Carb Breakfast Options

1. Avocado and Egg Breakfast Bowl

- Ingredients:

- 1 avocado, diced

- 2 eggs, poached or scrambled

- 1/2 cup cherry tomatoes, halved

- 1/4 cup feta cheese

- 1 tablespoon olive oil

- Salt and pepper to taste

- Instructions:

1. Arrange avocado, eggs, and cherry tomatoes in a bowl.

2. Sprinkle with feta cheese and drizzle with olive oil.

3. Season with salt and pepper.

- Ingredients:

-/4 cup chia seeds

- 1 cup unsweetened almond milk

- 1 tablespoon maple syrup

- 1/2 teaspoon vanilla extract

- Toppings: fresh berries, nuts, coconut flakes

- Instructions:

1. Combine chia seeds, almond milk, maple syrup, and vanilla extract in a jar.

2. Stir well and refrigerate overnight.

3. Top with fresh berries, nuts, and coconut flakes before serving.

Lunch Recipes

High-Carb Lunch Options

1. Chicken and Brown Rice Buddha Bowl

- Ingredients:

- 1 cup cooked brown rice

- 4 oz grilled chicken breast, sliced

- 1/2 cup steamed broccoli

- 1/2 cup roasted sweet potato cubes

- 1/4 cup shredded carrots

- 1 tablespoon tahini sauce

- Instructions:

1. Arrange brown rice, chicken, broccoli, sweet potato, and carrots in a bowl.

2. Drizzle with tahini sauce.

- Ingredients:

- 4 bell peppers, tops cut off and seeds removed

- 1 cup cooked quinoa

- 1/2 lb ground turkey

- 1/2 cup black beans

- 1/2 cup corn

- 1/4 cup diced tomatoes

- 1/4 cup shredded cheese

- Instructions:

1. Preheat oven to 375°F (190°C).

2. Brown ground turkey in a skillet.

3. Mix quinoa, black beans, corn, diced tomatoes, and cooked turkey.

4. Stuff bell peppers with the mixture and top with shredded cheese.

5. Bake for 25-30 minutes, until the peppers are tender.

Low-Carb Lunch Options

1. Shrimp and Avocado Salad

- Ingredients:

- 4 oz cooked shrimp

- 1 avocado, diced

- 2 cups mixed greens

- 1/4 cup cherry tomatoes, halved

- 1/4 cup cucumber, sliced

- 2 tablespoons olive oil

- 1 tablespoon lemon juice

- Salt and pepper to taste

- Instructions:

1. Toss mixed greens, avocado, cherry tomatoes, and cucumber in a bowl.

2. Top with cooked shrimp.

3. Drizzle with olive oil and lemon juice, and season with salt and pepper.

2. Zucchini Noodles with Pesto and Grilled Chicken

- Ingredients:

- 2 medium zucchinis, spiralized

- 4 oz grilled chicken breast, sliced

- 2 tablespoons pesto sauce

- 1 tablespoon pine nuts

- 1/4 cup cherry tomatoes, halved

- Instructions:

1. Sauté zucchini noodles in a skillet for 2-3 minutes until tender.

2. Toss with pesto sauce.

3. Top with grilled chicken, pine nuts, and cherry tomatoes.

Chapter 5: Exercise and Carb Cycling

Carb cycling is a powerful strategy for managing weight and enhancing athletic performance. However, to maximize its benefits, it's crucial to pair it with an effective exercise regimen. This chapter will explore the importance of exercise in weight loss, various types of workouts, how to align these workouts with your carb cycling plan, and sample workout routines for high-carb and low-carb days. We'll also cover the importance of rest and recovery in your overall fitness journey.

The Importance of Exercise in Weight Loss

Exercise is a cornerstone of a successful weight loss program, and its benefits extend far beyond simply burning calories. Here's why exercise is crucial in a carb cycling plan:

1. Boosts Metabolic Rate

- Regular exercise, particularly strength training, increases muscle mass. Muscle tissue burns more calories at rest compared to fat tissue, thus boosting your basal metabolic rate (BMR).

2. Enhances Fat Loss

- Exercise helps create a caloric deficit, which is necessary for fat loss. Combining this with carb cycling can optimize fat burning, particularly on low-carb days when the body is more reliant on fat for fuel.

3. Improves Insulin Sensitivity

- Physical activity enhances insulin sensitivity, meaning your muscles can better utilize glucose for energy. This is particularly beneficial on high-carb days, as it helps prevent excessive insulin spikes and promotes glycogen storage.

4. Preserves Lean Muscle Mass

- While losing weight, it's essential to preserve lean muscle mass to maintain metabolic rate and overall strength. Strength training is especially effective at preserving muscle during a calorie deficit.

5. Enhances Cardiovascular Health

- Cardiovascular exercises, such as running, cycling, and swimming, improve heart health, increase lung capacity, and reduce the risk of chronic diseases like hypertension and diabetes.

6. Boosts Mental Health

- Exercise releases endorphins, which can reduce stress, anxiety, and depression, enhancing overall mental well-being and motivation.

Types of Workouts: Cardio, Strength Training, and Flexibility

To create a balanced exercise routine, it's important to include various types of workouts: cardio, strength training, and flexibility exercises.

1. Cardiovascular Workouts

Cardiovascular, or aerobic, exercises involve sustained physical activity that raises your heart rate and improves the efficiency of your cardiovascular system. These workouts are effective for burning calories and improving endurance.

- **Examples:** Running, cycling, swimming, brisk walking, rowing, and group fitness classes.

- **Benefits:** Improved heart health, increased lung capacity, enhanced stamina, and effective calorie burning.

2. Strength Training Workouts

Strength training, or resistance training, focuses on building muscle mass and strength. This can involve lifting weights, using resistance bands, or performing bodyweight exercises.

- **Examples:** Weightlifting, bodyweight exercises (push-ups, squats, lunges), resistance band workouts, and machine-based exercises.

- **Benefits:** Increased muscle mass, enhanced metabolic rate, improved bone density, and better functional strength.

3. Flexibility and Mobility Workouts

Flexibility and mobility exercises aim to improve the range of motion of your joints and muscles. These workouts are crucial for preventing injuries and enhancing overall movement efficiency.

- **Examples:** Stretching routines, yoga, Pilates, and dynamic warm-ups.

- **Benefits:** Improved flexibility, reduced risk of injuries, enhanced posture, and greater ease of movement.

How to Pair Workouts with Your Carb Cycling Plan

Aligning your workouts with your carb cycling plan can optimize performance and recovery. Here's how to strategically pair different types of workouts with high-carb and low-carb days:

1. High-Carb Days

High-carb days are designed to provide ample energy for intense workouts and aid in muscle recovery. On these days, your body benefits from the increased glycogen stores provided by higher carbohydrate intake.

- Ideal Workouts:

- **Intense Cardio Sessions:** Long-distance running, high-intensity interval training (HIIT), and spinning classes.

- **Heavy Strength Training:** Compound lifts such as squats, deadlifts, bench presses, and powerlifting routines.

- **Endurance Activities:** Marathon training, long bike rides, and swimming sessions.

2. Low-Carb Days

Low-carb days aim to promote fat oxidation and enhance metabolic flexibility. Since glycogen stores are lower, workouts on these days should be less intense to prevent excessive fatigue and muscle breakdown.

- Ideal Workouts:

- **Low-Intensity Cardio:** Walking, light jogging, steady-state cycling, and swimming.

- **Moderate Strength Training:** Bodyweight exercises, resistance band workouts, and lighter weightlifting with higher repetitions.

- **Flexibility and Mobility Workouts:** Yoga, stretching routines, and Pilates to improve flexibility and aid in recovery.

Sample Workout Routines

To help you integrate exercise effectively into your carb cycling plan, here are sample workout routines for high-carb and low-carb days:

High-Carb Day Workouts

1. Intense Cardio and Strength Training Session

- Warm-Up:

- 10 minutes of dynamic stretching (leg swings, arm circles, torso twists)

- 5 minutes of light jogging or jumping jacks

- Cardio:

- HIIT on the treadmill: 30 seconds sprint, 60 seconds walking (repeat 10 times)

- Strength Training:

- Squats: 4 sets of 8-10 reps

- Deadlifts: 4 sets of 8-10 reps

- Bench Press: 4 sets of 8-10 reps

- Bent Over Rows: 4 sets of 8-10 reps

- Shoulder Press: 3 sets of 10-12 reps

- Bicep Curls: 3 sets of 12-15 reps

- Tricep Dips: 3 sets of 12-15 reps

- Cool-Down:

- 5-10 minutes of static stretching (hamstring stretch, quad stretch, chest stretch)

2. Endurance Training

- Warm-Up:

- 10 minutes of light jogging and dynamic stretches

- Endurance Workout:

- Long-distance run (10-15 km at a moderate pace)

- Cool-Down:

- 5-10 minutes of walking followed by static stretching

Low-Carb Day Workout

1. Low-Intensity Cardio and Bodyweight Training

- Warm-Up:

- 5 minutes of light walking and dynamic stretches

- Cardio:

- 30-45 minutes of brisk walking or light jogging

- Bodyweight Strength Training:

- Push-Ups: 3 sets of 15-20 reps

- Bodyweight Squats: 3 sets of 15-20 reps

- Lunges: 3 sets of 12-15 reps per leg

- Plank: 3 sets of 60 seconds

- Glute Bridges: 3 sets of 15-20 reps

- Cool-Down:

- 5-10 minutes of static stretching focusing on major muscle groups

2. Flexibility and Mobility Routine

- Warm-Up:

- 5 minutes of light cardio (walking or jogging)

- Yoga Session:

- 30-45 minutes of yoga, focusing on poses that improve flexibility and mobility (downward dog, warrior poses, child's pose)

- Cool-Down:

- 5-10 minutes of deep breathing and meditation

Rest and Recovery

Rest and recovery are integral to any fitness program, particularly when following a carb cycling plan. Proper recovery ensures that your muscles repair and grow, preventing injuries and promoting overall well-being.

1. The Importance of Rest Days

Rest days allow your muscles to recover from the stress of intense workouts. Without adequate rest, you risk overtraining, which can lead to fatigue, decreased performance, and injuries.

- **Benefits:** Enhanced muscle recovery, reduced risk of injuries, improved performance, and mental rejuvenation.

2. Active Recovery

Active recovery involves engaging in low-intensity activities on rest days to promote blood flow and aid in muscle repair without the strain of intense exercise.

- **Examples:** Light walking, gentle yoga, stretching, or casual swimming.

3. Sleep

Sleep is a critical component of recovery. During deep sleep, the body releases growth hormone, which is essential for muscle repair and growth.

- Tips for Better Sleep:

- **Maintain a consistent sleep schedule.**

- Create a restful environment (dark, cool, and quiet).

- Avoid caffeine and electronic devices before bed.

- Practice relaxation techniques like meditation or deep breathing.

4. Nutrition for Recovery

Proper nutrition supports recovery by providing the necessary nutrients for muscle repair and replenishment of glycogen stores.

- **Protein:** Essential for muscle repair. Include high-quality protein sources in your post-workout meals.

- **Carbohydrates:** Help replenish glycogen stores, especially after intense workouts. Pair with protein for optimal recovery.

- **Hydration:** Stay hydrated to support muscle function and overall recovery. Drink water throughout the day and consider electrolyte drinks post-exercise.

5. Stretching and Foam Rolling

Incorporating stretching and foam rolling into your routine can help reduce muscle soreness and improve flexibility.

- **Stretching:** Focus on static stretching after workouts to improve flexibility and aid in muscle recovery.

- **Foam Rolling:** Use a foam roller to massage and release tight muscles, enhancing blood flow.

Chapter 6: The 21-Day Plan

Embarking on a 21-day carb cycling plan can set the foundation for long-term success in achieving your health and fitness goals. This chapter provides a comprehensive guide to help you get started, build momentum, and adjust the plan to suit your lifestyle. Each week will have detailed daily meal plans and workout routines tailored for high-carb and low-carb days, ensuring a balanced approach to nutrition and exercise.

Week 1: Getting Started

The first week is all about establishing a routine and familiarizing yourself with the carb-cycling principles. You'll alternate between high-carb and low-carb days to kickstart your metabolism and adjust your body to this new way of eating and exercising.

Meal Plan:

- **Breakfast:Greek Yogurt Parfait**

- **1 cup Greek yogurt**

- **1/2 cup granola**

- **1/2 cup mixed berries**

- **1 tablespoon honey**

- **Snack:Apple with Almond Butter**

- **1 apple, sliced**

- 2 tablespoons almond butter

- Lunch: Quinoa and Chickpea Salad

- 1 cup cooked quinoa

- 1/2 cup chickpeas

- 1/4 cup diced cucumbers

- 1/4 cup cherry tomatoes

- 2 tablespoons feta cheese

- 1 tablespoon olive oil

- 1 tablespoon lemon juice

- Snack: Hummus and Veggie Sticks

- 1/2 cup hummus

- Assorted vegetable sticks (carrots, celery, bell peppers)

- Dinner: Baked Salmon with Sweet Potato and Asparagus

- 6 oz baked salmon

- 1 medium sweet potato, baked

- 1 cup roasted asparagus

- 1 tablespoon olive oil

Workout Plan:

- **Warm-Up:**

- 10 minutes of dynamic stretching (leg swings, arm circles, torso twists)

- 5 minutes of light jogging or jumping jacks

- **Cardio:**

- HIIT on the treadmill: 30 seconds sprint, 60 seconds walking (repeat 10 times)

- **Strength Training:**

- Squats: 4 sets of 8-10 reps

- Deadlifts: 4 sets of 8-10 reps

- Bench Press: 4 sets of 8-10 reps

- Bent Over Rows: 4 sets of 8-10 reps

- Shoulder Press: 3 sets of 10-12 reps

- Bicep Curls: 3 sets of 12-15 reps

- Tricep Dips: 3 sets of 12-15 reps

- Cool-Down:

- 5-10 minutes of static stretching (hamstring stretch, quad stretch, chest stretch)

Day 2: Low-Carb Day

Meal Plan:

- Breakfast: Spinach and Mushroom Omelette

- 3 eggs

- 1 cup spinach

- 1/2 cup mushrooms, sliced

- 1/4 cup shredded cheese

- Snack: Greek Yogurt with Chia Seeds

- 1 cup Greek yogurt

- 1 tablespoon chia seeds

- Lunch: Grilled Chicken Salad

- 4 oz grilled chicken breast

- Mixed greens

- 1/4 cup cherry tomatoes

- 1/4 avocado, sliced

- 2 tablespoons olive oil

- 1 tablespoon balsamic vinegar

- Snack: Cheese and Nuts

- 1 oz cheese (cheddar, mozzarella)

- 1/4 cup mixed nuts

- Dinner: Beef Stir-Fry with Broccoli and Bell Peppers

- 6 oz lean beef strips

- 1 cup broccoli florets

- 1/2 cup bell peppers, sliced

- 2 tablespoons soy sauce

- 1 tablespoon olive oil

Workout Plan:

- Warm-Up:

- 5 minutes of light walking and dynamic stretches

- Cardio:

- 30-45 minutes of brisk walking or light jogging

- Bodyweight Strength Training:

- Push-Ups: 3 sets of 15-20 reps

- Bodyweight Squats: 3 sets of 15-20 reps

- Lunges: 3 sets of 12-15 reps per leg

- Plank: 3 sets of 60 seconds

- Glute Bridges: 3 sets of 15-20 reps

- Cool-Down:

- 5-10 minutes of static stretching focusing on major muscle groups

Day 3: High-Carb Day

Meal Plan:

- Breakfast: Oatmeal with Banana and Peanut Butter

- 1/2 cup rolled oats

- 1 cup water or milk

- 1 banana, sliced

- 1 tablespoon peanut butter

- 1 teaspoon honey

- 1/2 teaspoon cinnamon

- Snack: Smoothie Bowl

- 1 banana, frozen

- 1/2 cup mixed berries, frozen

- 1/2 cup Greek yogurt

- 1/2 cup almond milk

- Toppings: granola, chia seeds, fresh berries

- Lunch: Chicken and Brown Rice Buddha Bowl

- 1 cup cooked brown rice

- 4 oz grilled chicken breast, sliced

- 1/2 cup steamed broccoli

- 1/2 cup roasted sweet potato cubes

- 1/4 cup shredded carrots

- 1 tablespoon tahini sauce

- Snack: Greek Yogurt with Mixed Nuts

- 1 cup Greek yogurt

- 1/4 cup mixed nuts

- Dinner: Turkey and Quinoa Stuffed Peppers

- 4 bell peppers, tops cut off and seeds removed

- 1 cup cooked quinoa

- 1/2 lb ground turkey

- 1/2 cup black beans

- 1/2 cup corn

- 1/4 cup diced tomatoes

- 1/4 cup shredded cheese

Workout Plan:

- Warm-Up:

- 10 minutes of light jogging and dynamic stretches

- Cardio:

- Long-distance run (10-15 km at a moderate pace)

- Cool-Down:

- 5-10 minutes of walking followed by static stretching

Day 4: Low-Carb Day

Meal Plan:

- **Breakfast: Avocado and Egg Breakfast Bowl**

- 1 avocado, diced

- 2 eggs, poached or scrambled

- 1/2 cup cherry tomatoes, halved

- 1/4 cup feta cheese

- 1 tablespoon olive oil

- Salt and pepper to taste

- **Snack: Chia Pudding**

- 1/4 cup chia seeds

- 1 cup unsweetened almond milk

- 1 tablespoon maple syrup

- 1/2 teaspoon vanilla extract

- Toppings: fresh berries, nuts, coconut flakes

- Lunch: Shrimp and Avocado Salad

- 4 oz cooked shrimp

- 1 avocado, diced

- 2 cups mixed greens

- 1/4 cup cherry tomatoes, halved

- 1/4 cup cucumber, sliced

- 2 tablespoons olive oil

- 1 tablespoon lemon juice

- Salt and pepper to taste

- Snack: Cheese and Nuts

- 1 oz cheese (cheddar, mozzarella)

- 1/4 cup mixed nuts

- Dinner: Zucchini Noodles with Pesto and Grilled Chicken

- 2 medium zucchinis, spiralized

- 4 oz grilled chicken breast, sliced

- 2 tablespoons pesto sauce

- 1 tablespoon pine nuts

- 1/4 cup cherry tomatoes, halved

Workout Plan:

- Warm-Up:

- 5 minutes of light cardio (walking or jogging)

- Yoga Session:

- 30-45 minutes of yoga, focusing on poses that improve flexibility and mobility (downward dog, warrior poses, child's pose)

- Cool-Down:

- 5-10 minutes of deep breathing and meditation

Day 5: High-Carb Day Meal Plan:

- **Breakfast: Smoothie Bowl**

- 1 banana, frozen

- 1/2 cup mixed berries, frozen

- 1/2 cup Greek yogurt

- 1/2 cup almond milk

- Toppings: granola, chia seeds, fresh berries

- Snack: Apple with Almond Butter

- 1 apple, sliced

- 2 tablespoons almond butter

- **Lunch:** Quinoa and Chickpea Salad

- 1 cup cooked quinoa

- 1/2 cup chickpeas

- 1/4 cup diced cucumbers

- 1/4 cup cherry tomatoes

- 2 tablespoons feta cheese

- 1 tablespoon olive oil

- 1 tablespoon lemon juice

- Snack: Hummus and Veggie Sticks

- 1/2 cup hummus

- Assorted vegetable sticks (carrots, celery, bell peppers)

- Dinner:Baked Salmon with Sweet Potato and Asparagus

- 6 oz baked salmon

- 1 medium sweet potato, baked

Chapter 7: Overcoming Challenges

Embarking on a carb cycling journey is an effective way to manage weight, enhance fitness, and improve overall health. However, like any lifestyle change, it comes with its own set of challenges. This chapter aims to address these challenges and provide strategies to overcome them. From dealing with cravings and staying motivated to managing social situations and special occasions, hitting plateaus, and ensuring long-term maintenance and lifestyle changes, this comprehensive guide will help you stay on track and achieve your goals.

Dealing with Cravings

Cravings can be one of the most difficult challenges to overcome when following a carb cycling plan. Here are some strategies to help manage and mitigate them:

1. Identify the Source of Cravings

- Cravings can be triggered by a variety of factors, including emotional stress, boredom, or nutritional deficiencies. Understanding the root cause can help you address it more effectively.

2. Stay Hydrated

- **Sometimes, wha**t feels like a craving might be thirst. Drink plenty of water throughout the day to stay hydrated and help reduce the intensity of cravings.

3. Eat Regularly

- Skipping meals or going too long without eating can lead to intense hunger and cravings. Aim to eat balanced meals and snacks at regular intervals to maintain stable blood sugar levels.

4. Include Protein and Fiber in Your Diet

- Protein and fiber-rich foods can help you feel fuller for longer, reducing the likelihood of cravings. Include sources of lean protein (chicken, fish, tofu) and fiber (vegetables, fruits, whole grains) in your meals.

5. Allow Yourself Occasional Treats

- Completely depriving yourself of certain foods can backfire, leading to binge eating. Allow yourself occasional treats in moderation to satisfy your cravings without derailing your progress.

6. Keep Healthy Snacks on Hand

- Having healthy snacks readily available can help you resist the temptation to reach for unhealthy options. Nuts, seeds, fruit, and yogurt are excellent choices for curbing cravings.

7. Distract Yourself

- Cravings often pass if you can distract yourself. Engage in activities such as going for a walk, reading a book, or calling a friend to take your mind off food.

Staying Motivated

Maintaining motivation over the long term can be challenging. Here are some tips to keep you inspired and committed to your carb-cycling journey:

1. Set Clear Goals

- Establish both short-term and long-term goals. Make them specific, measurable, achievable, relevant, and time-bound (SMART). For example, aim to lose 5 pounds in a month or run a 5k in six weeks.

2. Track Your Progress

- Keep a journal or use an app to track your meals, workouts, and progress. Seeing your achievements in black and white can be incredibly motivating.

3. Find a Support System

- Surround yourself with supportive friends and family or join a community of like-minded individuals. Sharing your journey with others can provide encouragement and accountability.

4. Reward Yourself

- Celebrate your milestones with non-food rewards, such as a new workout outfit, a spa day, or a fun outing. Recognizing your achievements can boost your motivation to keep going.

5. Stay Positive

- Focus on the positive changes you're making and the benefits you're experiencing. A positive mindset can help you stay motivated and overcome obstacles.

6. Mix Things Up

- Avoid monotony by varying your workouts and meal plans. Trying new exercises and recipes can keep things interesting and prevent burnout.

7. Visualize Your Success

- Take a few minutes each day to visualize yourself achieving your goals. Picture yourself healthier, fitter, and happier. This mental practice can reinforce your commitment and drive.

Managing Social Situations and Special Occasions

Social situations and special occasions often involve food and drink, which can be challenging when sticking to a carb cycling plan. Here are strategies to help you navigate these events without feeling deprived or left out:

1. Plan Ahead

- If you know you're going to a social event, plan your meals and workouts around it. Adjust your carb intake and ensure you have healthy options available.

2. Communicate Your Goals

- Let friends and family know about your goals and ask for their support. Most people will respect your choices and may even offer healthier options.

3. Bring a Healthy Dish

- If you're attending a potluck or gathering, bring a healthy dish that aligns with your plan. This ensures you have something nutritious to eat and can share with others.

4. Focus on Socializing

- Shift your focus from food to socializing. Engage in conversations, participate in activities, and enjoy the company of others. This can help distract you from food temptations.

5. Make Smart Choices

- At events, look for healthier options such as vegetables, lean proteins, and salads. Avoid heavy, carb-laden dishes, and practice portion control if you indulge in treats.

6. Limit Alcohol

- Alcohol can add empty calories and lower your inhibitions, leading to overeating. If you choose to drink, do so in moderation and opt for lower-calorie options like wine or spirits with soda water.

7. Don't Be Too Hard on Yourself

- If you indulge more than planned, don't beat yourself up. One meal or event won't derail your progress. Get back on track with your next meal and workout.

When You Hit a Plateau

Hitting a plateau can be frustrating, but it's a common part of any weight loss or fitness journey. Here are strategies to break through and continue making progress:

1. Reassess Your Goals

- Evaluate your current goals and progress. Are your goals still realistic and achievable? Adjust them if necessary to reflect your current situation and progress.

2. Change Up Your Routine

- Your body can adapt to the same workout and meal plans, leading to plateaus. Introduce new exercises, increase the intensity of your workouts, or change your carb cycling pattern to keep your body guessing.

3. Monitor Your Intake

- Ensure you're accurately tracking your food intake. Small inaccuracies can add up and affect your progress. Use a food journal or app to keep detailed records.

4. Increase Protein Intake

- Higher protein intake can boost metabolism, support muscle growth, and keep you feeling fuller longer. Incorporate lean protein sources into each meal.

5. Adjust Caloric Intake

- As you lose weight, your caloric needs decrease. Recalculate your daily caloric needs and adjust your intake accordingly to continue losing weight.

6. Get Enough Sleep

- Lack of sleep can hinder weight loss and overall progress. Aim for 7-9 hours of quality sleep per night to support recovery and metabolic function.

7. Stay Hydrated

- Dehydration can slow metabolism and affect performance. Drink plenty of water throughout the day to stay hydrated and support your weight loss efforts.

Long-Term Maintenance and Lifestyle Changes

The ultimate goal of any weight loss or fitness plan is to create sustainable habits that lead to long-term health and well-being. Here are strategies for maintaining your progress and making lasting lifestyle changes:

1. Adopt a Balanced Approach

- While carb cycling can be effective for weight loss and muscle gain, it's important to find a balance that you can maintain long-term. Incorporate a variety of foods and allow flexibility in your diet.

2. Continue Tracking

- Even after reaching your goals, continue tracking your food intake and workouts to stay accountable. This can help you maintain your progress and make adjustments as needed.

3. Stay Active

- Regular physical activity is crucial for long-term health. Find activities you enjoy and make them a part of your routine. Aim for a mix of cardio, strength training, and flexibility exercises.

4. Prioritize Nutrition

- Focus on nutrient-dense foods that provide vitamins, minerals, and other essential nutrients. Limit processed foods, sugary drinks, and excessive unhealthy fats.

5. Manage Stress

- Chronic stress can negatively impact your health and weight. Practice stress management techniques such as meditation, deep breathing, and regular physical activity.

6. Build a Support System

- Surround yourself with supportive friends, family, or a community of like-minded individuals. Having a support system can provide encouragement, accountability, and motivation.

7. Continue Learning

- Stay informed about nutrition, fitness, and health trends. Read books, attend workshops, and seek advice from experts to keep your knowledge up-to-date.

8. Set New Goals

- Once you've achieved your initial goals, set new ones to keep yourself challenged and motivated. This could be a new fitness milestone, learning a new skill, or improving another aspect of your health.

9. Practice Mindful Eating

- Pay attention to your hunger and fullness cues, and avoid emotional eating. Mindful eating can help you maintain a healthy relationship with food and prevent overeating.

10. Be Kind to Yourself

- Remember that setbacks and challenges are a normal part of any journey. Be kind to yourself, learn from your experiences, and stay focused on your long-term health and well-being.

Chapter 8: Success Stories and Testimonials

Success stories and testimonials serve as powerful motivators, offering real-life proof of what is achievable through dedication and perseverance. In this chapter, you will find inspiring accounts of real-life transformations, practical tips from successful carb cyclers, and motivational quotes that can fuel your journey.

Real-Life Transformations

Emily's Journey: From Overweight to Athletes

Emily had always struggled with her weight. At her heaviest, she felt sluggish, uncomfortable in her skin, and lacked confidence. Determined to change, she stumbled upon carb cycling. The concept intrigued her: alternating between high-carb and low-carb days seemed manageable and less restrictive than other diets she had tried.

Emily committed to a 21-day carb cycling plan. The first week was challenging as she adapted to the new eating pattern and integrated regular workouts into her routine. But she quickly noticed positive changes. Her energy levels increased, and the workouts became less daunting. By the end of the first month, she had lost 10 pounds and felt more vibrant than she had in years.

Motivated by her initial success, Emily continued carb cycling, incorporating more complex workouts and fine-tuning her nutrition. Within six months, she had shed 40 pounds and transformed her body composition. Emily didn't just lose weight; she built muscle, improved her cardiovascular health, and regained her confidence. Today, she participates in athletic events, including marathons and triathlons, and has become an inspiration to her friends and family.

John's Transformation: Overcoming a Plateau

John was an avid gym-goer who had always maintained a reasonably healthy diet. However, despite his efforts, he hit a weight loss plateau that lasted for months. Frustrated, he decided to try carb cycling, hoping to reignite his progress.

John's approach was meticulous. He meticulously planned his high-carb and low-carb days around his workout schedule, ensuring that he had enough energy for intense training sessions. He also focused on nutrient timing, consuming most of his carbs around his workouts to maximize muscle glycogen replenishment and recovery.

The results were swift and impressive. Within a few weeks, John broke through his plateau and started losing weight again. His muscle definition improved, and he felt stronger and more energized during his workouts. By the end of three months, John had not only reached his goal weight but also achieved a level of fitness he hadn't thought possible. Carb cycling, coupled with strategic exercise, had transformed his body and reignited his passion for fitness.

Samantha's Story: Balancing Family Life and Fitness

As a busy mother of three, Samantha found it challenging to prioritize her health. Her days were filled with work, family responsibilities, and household chores, leaving little time for herself. She often resorted to quick, unhealthy meals and felt constantly fatigued.

Determined to make a change, Samantha decided to try carb cycling. She saw it as a flexible approach that could fit into her hectic schedule. She started by preparing meal plans that included family-friendly, carb-cycling recipes. She also scheduled short, high-intensity workouts that could be done at home.

The first few weeks were tough, but Samantha soon found a rhythm. She involved her family in her journey, encouraging healthy eating habits for everyone. The results were life-changing. Samantha lost weight, gained energy, and felt more present and engaged with her family. Her transformation wasn't just physical; it was emotional and mental. She felt empowered and proud of the example she was setting for her children.

Tips from Successful Carb Cyclers

Emily's Tips:

1. **Meal Prep is Key:** Emily emphasizes the importance of meal prep. "Planning and preparing your meals in advance ensures you stay on track, especially on busy days."

2. **Stay Hydrated:** "Drink plenty of water. It helps control and keeps your body functioning optimally."

3. **Listen to Your Body:** "Adjust your carb intake based on how you feel. If you're extremely active, you might need more carbs even on low-carb days."

John's Tips:

1. Track Your Progress: "Keep a detailed log of your meals, workouts, and how you feel each day. This can help you make necessary adjustments and stay motivated."

2. Nutrient Timing: "Consume the majority of your carbs around your workouts. This helps with energy and recovery."

3. Stay Consistent: "Consistency is more important than perfection. Stick with the plan, and results will follow."

Samantha's Tips:

1. Involve Your Family: "Make healthy eating a family affair. It's easier to stick to your plan when everyone is on board."

2. Find Short, Effective Workouts: "High-intensity interval training (HIIT) can be done in a short amount of time and is very effective."

3. Be Flexible: "Life happens. If you have a bad day, don't stress. Just get back on track the next day."

Inspirational Quotes and Motivations

Emotional quotes can serve as a daily reminder of your goals and help keep you motivated. Here are some powerful quotes to inspire you on your carb-cycling journey:

**1. "The journey of a thousand miles begins with one step."
– Lao Tzu**

- This quote emphasizes the importance of starting, no matter how daunting the journey might seem.

2. Believe you can and you're halfway there." – Theodore Roosevelt

- Belief in your ability to succeed is crucial. This mindset can propel you forward even on challenging days.

3. "Success is not final, failure is not fatal: It is the courage to continue that count." – Winston Churchill

- Persistence is key. Embrace both successes and setbacks as part of your journey.

4. "What you get by achieving your goals is not as important as what you become by achieving your goals." – Zig Ziglar

- The transformation process is about personal growth and becoming the best version of yourself.

5. "You don't have to be great to start, but you have to start to be great." – Zig Ziglar

- Taking the first step, no matter how small, is essential to achieving greatness.

6. "It's not about perfect. It's about effort. And when you bring that effort every single day, that's where transformation happens. That's how change occurs." – Jillian Michaels

- Consistent effort is more important than perfection. Keep pushing forward every day.

7. "Your body can stand almost anything. It's your mind that you have to convince." – Unknown

- Mental strength and determination are critical in overcoming physical challenges.

8. "The only bad workout is the one that didn't happen." – Unknown

- Every workout counts. Even if it's not perfect, showing up is what matters.

9. "Take care of your body. It's the only place you have to live." – Jim Rohn

- Prioritizing your health is an investment in your future.

10. "Discipline is the bridge between goals and accomplishment." – Jim Rohn

- Discipline and consistency are essential for reaching your goals.

Final Thoughts

The stories, tips, and quotes shared in this chapter illustrate that success in carb cycling, and any fitness or health journey, is achievable with the right mindset, strategies, and support. Whether you're just starting or looking for ways to overcome challenges, these real-life transformations and words of wisdom can inspire and guide you.

Remember that everyone's journey is unique. What works for one person might need to be adjusted for another. Stay committed, be patient, and don't be afraid to seek support and advice along the way. Your transformation is not just about reaching a specific weight or fitness goal but about embracing a healthier, more balanced lifestyle.

By learning from those who have successfully navigated the challenges of carb cycling, you can apply their insights to your journey. Use their experiences as motivation to keep pushing forward, even when the going gets tough. Celebrate your progress, no matter how small, and keep your eyes on the bigger picture: a healthier, happier you.

Your carb cycling journey is not just a diet or a fitness plan—it's a path to self-improvement and empowerment. With the tools, strategies, and inspiration provided in this chapter, you're well-equipped to overcome any challenges that come your way and achieve lasting success.

Chapter 9: Resources

The journey to a healthier and fitter lifestyle is made easier with the right resources at your fingertips. In this chapter, we'll explore a wealth of resources including recommended reading, useful apps and websites, support groups and communities, and meal prep services and tools. These resources can provide the information, support, and convenience you need to stay on track with your carb cycling plan and overall health goals.

Recommended Reading

Books are a valuable source of information and inspiration. Here are some highly recommended books that cover various aspects of nutrition, fitness, and wellness, providing a deeper understanding and practical advice for your carb cycling journey.

1. "The Carb Cycling Diet: Optimize Your Health and Performance with Carb Cycling" by Jay Robb

- This book offers a comprehensive guide to carb cycling, detailing how to balance your intake of carbohydrates to enhance fat loss and muscle gain. Robb provides practical meal plans and recipes, making it easier to incorporate carb cycling into your lifestyle.

2. "The Science of Nutrition" by Rhiannon Lambert

- Lambert's book breaks down complex nutritional science into easy-to-understand concepts. It covers the roles of different macronutrients and micronutrients, helping you make informed choices about your diet.

3. "The New Rules of Lifting for Women" by Lou Schuler, Cassandra Forsythe, and Alwyn Cosgrove

- This book is an excellent resource for women looking to incorporate strength training into their fitness routines. It offers detailed workout plans and emphasizes the importance of combining proper nutrition with exercise for optimal results.

4. "Atomic Habits: An Easy & Proven Way to Build Good Habits & Break Bad Ones" by James Clear

- While not specifically about carb cycling, Clear's book provides valuable insights into habit formation. Understanding how to build and maintain healthy habits can be a game-changer in your fitness and nutrition journey.

5. "Burn the Fat, Feed the Muscle: Transform Your Body Forever Using the Secrets of the Leanest People in the World" by Tom Venuto

- Venuto's book offers a holistic approach to body transformation, combining diet, exercise, and mindset. It includes practical tips on how to cycle carbs for fat loss and muscle gain.

6. "The Complete Guide to Sports Nutrition" by Anita Bean

- This book is a thorough guide to sports nutrition, covering everything from meal planning to hydration strategies. It's an excellent resource for those looking to optimize their diet for athletic performance.

7. "Intuitive Eating: A Revolutionary Anti-Diet Approach" by Evelyn Tribole and Elyse Resch

- For those who have struggled with restrictive diets, this book offers a different perspective. It promotes a healthy relationship with food and encourages listening to your body's hunger and fullness cues.

8. "The Mindful Athlete: Secrets to Pure Performance" by George Mumford

- Mumford's book explores the mental aspects of athletic performance, emphasizing mindfulness and mental toughness. It's a great read for anyone looking to improve their focus and resilience.

Useful Apps and Websites

Technology can be a powerful ally in your health and fitness journey. Here are some apps and websites that can help you track your progress, find workout plans, and stay informed about nutrition.

1. MyFitnessPal

- Description: A comprehensive app for tracking your food intake and exercise.

- Features: Extensive food database, barcode scanner, nutrient tracking, integration with fitness trackers.

- Why It's Useful: MyFitnessPal makes it easy to log your meals and monitor your macronutrient intake, crucial for carb cycling.

2. Carb Manager

- Description: An app specifically designed for those following low-carb and ketogenic diets.

- Features: Macro tracking, meal planning, recipe database, shopping list generator.

- Why It's Useful: Carb Manager is ideal for tracking your carb intake and planning meals that fit into your carb cycling plan.

3. Fitbod

- Description: A personalized workout planning app.

- Features: Custom workout plans based on your goals, equipment, fitness level, exercise demonstrations, and progress tracking.

- Why It's Useful: Fitbod helps you design and track your workouts, ensuring you're making the most of your high-carb and low-carb days.

4. Lose It!

- Description: A user-friendly app for calorie counting and weight loss.

- Features: Food database, barcode scanner, macronutrient tracking, social features.

- Why It's Useful: Lose It! simplifies meal tracking and offers insights into your eating patterns, making it easier to stay on track with your carb cycling plan.

5. StrongLifts 5x5

- Description: A strength training app focusing on the 5x5 workout routine.

- Features: Workout logging, progress tracking, instructional videos, tips for improving form.

- Why It's Useful: StrongLifts 5x5 provides structured strength training routines, helping you build muscle and complement your carb cycling plan.

6. Healthline Nutrition

- Description: A website offering evidence-based articles on nutrition and wellness.

- Features: In-depth articles, meal plans, recipes, and expert advice.

- Why It's Useful: Healthline Nutrition is a reliable source of information, helping you make informed decisions about your diet and health.

7. Precision Nutrition

- Description: A website dedicated to providing science-based nutrition advice and coaching.

- Features: Articles, infographics, coaching programs, nutrition calculators.

- Why It's Useful: Precision Nutrition offers detailed, research-backed information on nutrition and fitness, perfect for those looking to delve deeper into their carb cycling journey.

8. Fitness Blender

- Description: A website offering free workout videos and fitness programs.

- Features: Hundreds of workout videos, customizable workout plans, and nutrition tips.

- Why It's Useful: Fitness Blender provides a variety of workouts, making it easy to find exercises that fit your schedule and goals.

Support Groups and Communities

Having a support system can make a significant difference in your success. Here are some online and offline communities where you can find encouragement, share experiences, and get advice.

1. Reddit - r/CarbCycling

- Description: A subreddit dedicated to carb cycling.

- Features: User-generated content, tips, success stories, Q&A.

- Why It's Useful: This community offers a wealth of practical advice and support from fellow carb cyclers.

2. MyFitnessPal Community

- Description: An online forum for users of the MyFitnessPal app.

- **Features:** Discussion boards, groups, challenges, success stories.

- Why It's Useful: The MyFitnessPal community provides a platform to connect with others, share tips, and stay motivated.

3. Facebook Groups

- Examples: "Carb Cycling Support Group," "Low Carb High Fat Success Stories"

- Features: Posts, discussions, live videos, events.

- Why It's Useful: Facebook groups offer a convenient way to engage with a community, ask questions, and share your journey.

4. Local Meetup Groups

- Description: In-person groups focused on health and fitness.

- Features: Group workouts, social events, workshops.

- Why It's Useful: Meetup groups provide face-to-face support and the opportunity to build friendships with like-minded individuals.

5. SparkPeople

- Description: An online health and fitness community.

- Features: Articles, forums, challenges, tracking tools.

- Why It's Useful: SparkPeople offers a comprehensive platform for tracking your progress and connecting with a supportive community.

6. Instagram Influencers

- Examples: @fitmencook, @thefitnesschef_, @keto.connect

- Features: Daily posts, stories, live sessions, Q&A.

- Why It's Useful: Following fitness and nutrition influencers can provide daily inspiration, tips, and motivation.

Meal Prep Services and Tools

Meal prep is a critical component of successful carb cycling. Here are some services and tools that can make meal planning and preparation easier.

1. Blue Apron

- Description: A meal kit delivery service.

- Features: Pre-portioned ingredients, step-by-step recipes, customizable plans.

- Why It's Useful: Blue Apron simplifies meal prep by providing all the ingredients and instructions you need to create healthy meals.

2. HelloFresh

- Description: A meal kit delivery service offering a variety of meal plans.

- Features: Fresh ingredients, easy-to-follow recipes, flexible subscriptions.

- Why It's Useful: HelloFresh offers diverse meal options, making it easy to find recipes that fit your carb cycling plan.

3. Meal Prep Containers

- Examples: Freshware, Prep Naturals, Fitpacker

- Features: Durable, microwave-safe, various sizes.

- Why It's Useful: High-quality meal prep containers make it easy to portion and store your meals, ensuring you stay on track with your nutrition.

4. Food Scale

- Examples: Etekcity, Ozeri, Greater Goods

- Features: Precise measurements, tare function, digital display.

- Why It's Useful: A food scale helps you accurately measure your food portions, crucial for tracking your macronutrient intake.

5. Slow Cooker/Instant Pot

- Examples: Crock-Pot, Instant Pot Duo, Ninja Foodi

- Features: Multiple cooking functions, programmable settings, large capacity.

- **Why It's Useful:** Slow cookers and Instant Pots allow for convenient, hands-off meal preparation, perfect for busy individuals.

6. Blender

- Examples: NutriBullet, Vitamix, Ninja

- Features: Powerful motors, multiple settings, durable blades.

- Why It's Useful: A good blender is essential for making smoothies, soups, and sauces, helping you incorporate more fruits and vegetables into your diet

Conclusion: Celebrating Your Success; Looking Forward: Maintaining a Healthy Lifestyle; Final Thoughts and Encouragement

As you conclude this book, it's time to reflect on the incredible journey you've undertaken. Completing the 21-day carb cycling plan is an achievement worthy of celebration. You've dedicated yourself to improving your health, and that deserves recognition. This chapter will help you celebrate your success, look forward to maintaining a healthy lifestyle, and leave you with some final thoughts and encouragement to continue your journey.

Celebrating Your Success

Your commitment to the 21-day carb cycling plan has led you to this moment. Whether you've lost weight, gained muscle, increased your energy levels, or simply developed a better understanding of your body's nutritional needs, your progress is significant.

1. Reflect on Your Achievements

Take a moment to reflect on where you started and where you are now. Consider keeping a journal to document your progress, including any physical changes, improved fitness levels, and shifts in your mindset. Reflecting on your achievements can reinforce the positive habits you've developed and motivate you to continue your healthy lifestyle.

2. Share Your Success

Sharing your journey with friends, family, or even on social media can be incredibly rewarding. It not only allows you to celebrate your accomplishments but also inspires others who may be struggling with their own health goals. Your story can be a powerful motivator for others to embark on their journey to better health.

3. Reward Yourself

Rewards can be a great way to acknowledge your hard work and dedication. Consider treating yourself to something special, whether it's a new workout outfit, a relaxing spa day, or a fun outing with friends. Rewarding yourself for your success reinforces positive behavior and encourages you to continue striving for your goals.

4. Set New Goals

While it's important to celebrate your current achievements, it's equally important to keep setting new goals to maintain your momentum. These goals can be related to fitness, nutrition, or personal growth. For example, you might aim to run a 5K, try a new sport, or learn more about nutrition and healthy cooking.

Looking Forward: Maintaining a Healthy Lifestyle

The 21-day carb cycling plan was just the beginning of your journey. Now, it's time to focus on maintaining the healthy habits you've developed and continuing to improve your overall well-being.

1. Continue Carb Cycling

Many people find carb cycling to be a sustainable and effective approach to maintaining their weight and energy levels. You can continue to cycle your carbs, adjusting the frequency and intensity based on your current fitness goals and lifestyle. Remember, flexibility is key. Don't be afraid to tweak your plan to suit your needs.

2. Embrace a Balanced Diet

While carb cycling can be an effective tool, it's important to maintain a balanced diet that includes a variety of nutrient-dense foods. Ensure that you're consuming adequate amounts of protein, healthy fats, and fiber-rich vegetables. A balanced diet supports overall health and helps you avoid nutritional deficiencies.

3. Keep Moving

Regular physical activity is crucial for maintaining a healthy lifestyle. Continue to incorporate a mix of cardio, strength training, and flexibility exercises into your routine. Aim to stay active most days of the week, and find activities that you enjoy to keep exercise fun and engaging.

4. Prioritize Mental Health

Your mental health is just as important as your physical health. Incorporate practices such as mindfulness, meditation, and stress management techniques into your daily routine. Taking care of your mental well-being can enhance your overall quality of life and help you stay motivated to maintain healthy habits.

5. Stay Hydrated

Adequate hydration is essential for optimal health. Make sure to drink plenty of water throughout the day, especially if you're active or live in a hot climate. Staying hydrated helps your body function properly and can improve your energy levels and cognitive function.

6. Get Enough Sleep

Quality sleep is vital for your health and well-being. Aim for 7-9 hours of sleep per night and establish a consistent sleep routine. Good sleep hygiene, such as avoiding screens before bedtime and creating a relaxing sleep environment, can improve the quality of your rest.

7. Continue Learning

The world of nutrition and fitness is always evolving. Stay informed by reading books, following reputable health websites, and seeking advice from qualified professionals. Continuing to educate yourself can help you make informed decisions about your health and keep you motivated to pursue new goals.

Final Thoughts and Encouragement

Embarking on a health and fitness journey is not always easy, but your dedication and perseverance have brought you this far. As you move forward, remember these key points to stay motivated and committed to your goals.

1. Embrace the Journey

Your health and fitness journey is a lifelong process. Embrace the ups and downs, and don't be discouraged by setbacks. Every step you take, no matter how small, brings you closer to your goals. Celebrate your progress, and remember that consistency is more important than perfection.

2. Find Your Why

Understanding your motivations can be a powerful tool for staying committed. Reflect on why you started this journey and what you hope to achieve. Whether it's improving your health, gaining confidence, or setting a positive example for loved ones, keeping your "why" in mind can help you stay focused and motivated.

3. Seek Support

Don't hesitate to seek support from friends, family, or health professionals. Surrounding yourself with a supportive community can provide encouragement, accountability, and valuable advice. Whether you join a fitness group, work with a nutritionist, or simply share your goals with a friend, support can make a significant difference in your success.

4. Be Kind to Yourself

Self-compassion is essential on your journey. Recognize that everyone has setbacks and challenges, and it's okay to make mistakes. Treat yourself with kindness and patience, and focus on the progress you've made rather than dwelling on any perceived failures.

5. Celebrate Every Victory

No matter how small, every victory is worth celebrating. Whether it's losing a pound, running an extra mile, or simply making a healthy meal choice, acknowledge your achievements. Celebrating your successes can boost your confidence and motivate you to keep going.

6. Stay Flexible

Life is full of unexpected changes and challenges. Stay flexible with your plans and be willing to adapt as needed. If you miss a workout or have an off day with your nutrition, don't be too hard on yourself. Adjust your plan and keep moving forward.

7. Focus on Long-Term Health

While short-term goals can be motivating, it's important to focus on long-term health and well-being. Aim to create sustainable habits that you can maintain for life. This approach not only leads to lasting results but also improves your overall quality of life.

8. Keep Your Eyes on the Prize

Remember why you started and what you hope to achieve. Keep your long-term goals in mind, and use them as motivation to stay committed to your healthy lifestyle. Visualize your success and let it drive you forward.

Conclusion

As you close this book, know that you have the tools, knowledge, and determination to continue your health and fitness journey. You've learned the science behind carb cycling, discovered practical strategies for meal planning and exercise, and gained insights from success stories and testimonials.

Your journey doesn't end here. It's an ongoing process of learning, growing, and striving for better health. Use the resources and support available to you, stay committed to your goals, and never stop believing in your ability to achieve great things.

Remember, the most important step is the one you're taking right now. Celebrate your progress, stay motivated, and keep moving forward. Your health and well-being are worth the effort, and you have the power to create the life you desire.

Thank you for choosing to embark on this journey with "21-Day Carb Cycling: Revitalize Your Body with Balanced Meals and Effective Workouts." Here's to your continued success and a lifetime of health and happiness.

www.ingramcontent.com/pod-product-compliance
Lightning Source LLC
Chambersburg PA
CBHW061637250726
48659CB00004B/1256